PHARMACOVIGILANCE DATABASE

Dr. Ravi Humbarwadi

www.gipv.net

Aris G, Oracle Argus, Empirica Trace, Sapphire, Clintrac are PV databases. This is a generic overview and gives a comprehensive idea of the different databases currently in use in pharmacovigilance across the globe.

An Oracle Argus specific overview is presented.

GENERAL SECTION

| Type of report | Country |

| First Received Date |

| Follow Up Received | Major |

If major TICK the tab

Type of report

There are various types of reports. Some of the report types are:

a. Spontaneous

b. Interventional Clinical Trial

c. Non-interventional Study (NIS)

d. Literature

e. Market research

f. Spontaneous literature

g. Spontaneous regulatory

Some advanced database fields for case processing are dependent on the type of report selected. For instance, if you select interventional clinical trial report as the type of report then further fields that open up may include blinding, unblinding, and SUSAR . These will not be available if you select the report type as spontaneous.

Country

This refers to the country where the event occurred.

First Received Date

Synonyms – Initial received date.

This is the first time that the sponsor (company) receives the ICSR from the reporter. Input the date, month and year.

Follow Up Received

A case may have several follow ups. As each follow up is received the date of receiving the follow up should be input.

Major

Each follow up can be categorized as major (synonym: significant) or minor (insignificant).

An addition of new event, outcomes of events, clinical progression, laboratory test results are examples of major follow up information.

Information such as batch numbers, affiliate numbers, manufacturers numbers are examples of minor follow up.

Tick tab – Major (significant) follow up

Untick tab – Minor (insignificant) follow up

STUDY DETAILS

Study Number	Site Number	Subject Number	Name of Study	Phase of study		Blinding	Blind Status

Study Description

Study Number

Input the study number and the subject number.

Site Number

Once the study number is entered, site number (synonym: center number) can be selected from a list. This list of center numbers is auto configured and is specific to the study number. A single multi-center study can have many site numbers. You need to select the site number reported in the source document.

Subject Number

Each participant in the study has a unique identification number. It is called the subject number. You need to input the subject number as reported in the source document.

Name of the study

The name of the study is auto-populated based on the study number.

Phase of the study

Input the study phase. It can be phase 1, 2, 3 or 4.

Blinding

The blinding is auto-populated based on the study number. It can be:

Open – label

Single Blind

Double Blind

Blinding Status

The blinding status refers to the whether the blind is broken. If the blind is broken then you can also input whether it has been broken by the sponsor or the investigator.

Study Description

The study description is auto-populated once the study number has been selected.

Example of study description: In study F0 1566 " A long term multicenter randomized interventional trial comparing the efficacy of Drug XX versus Drug YY in the subject with moderate to severe primary hypertension."

REPORTER DETAILS

First	Middle	Last

Healthcare professional

Occupation of the reporter

Organization

Postal Address

City	Province	Country

Email	Fax	Postal Code

All the above details pertain to the reporter (the person who has sent the case). In case you need to follow up for further details having all contact information of the reporter is essential.

Reporter's Name

Input the name of the reporter

Healthcare professional

Options: Yes, No and Unknown

Occupation of the reporter

Choose from dropdown

LITERATURE MODULE

Author	Title

Journal

Publication Date	Volume	Page

The above tabs are filled in to provide information in those case reports that are obtained from literature search.

In advanced software auto citation is facilitated.

The Vancouver citation is the preferred style of citation for medical and life sciences domain.

Below is the format of the Vancouver style.

Author: The names with initials appear first. The names are separated by comma. More than 1 initial is clubbed together. There is a full stop after all the names are listed.

Title: The title appears next. There is a full stop after the title.

Journal: The abbreviated name of the journal appears next.

Publication Date: This is followed by the year month and date.

Volume: Next comes the volume and issue number.

Page: And finally the page numbers.

See below the format examples of the literature citation.

For Journal Articles

- Rhease H, Billy CK, Pagliachi V. H_2-antihistamines: The anti-inflammatory actions and cardiac adverse effects. Blin Axp Allergy. 2003 Apr;52(3):386-93.

- Yachaguci B, Tamasaki J, Piero WL, Joisi U, Gondo I, Horita ET, et al. Inferior prognosis of surgery without chemotherapy for colon cancer. Asia J Surg Oncol. 2014 Jan 10;12(5):185. [Epub ahead of print]

PATIENT BASICS

First Name	Initial	Last Name

Initials

Patient Number

City	State	Country

Pincode

Address

Phone	Email

Private

The above is the patient information module for spontaneous cases.

Patient Name

The first name, initial of the patient and last name has to be input. This will get auto populated into the initials box.

However in view of patient confidentiality this field is seldom populated. Generally sponsors do not input the patient name but only the initials.

Initials

If no names are available but only initials are reported in the source document: Input in the initials box.

Generally the sponsors' may opt to input only the initials even if the patient name is available. This is done to protect the privacy and keep the case information confidential.

Patient number

Input patient number if reported.

Address

Name of the city, state and country of the patient to be entered as also the pin-code and postal address.

Private (Synonyms: Confidential, patient confidentiality, privacy tab)

Click this tab to keep the patient identity confidential.

The patient information helps to follow up with the patient for more details and to resolve queries. You can also contact the patient (with permission) for getting pending diagnosis, lab test results and causality of the event to the suspect drug or clinical progression of the events. This will result in a follow up report.

The below is the patient information module for clinical trial cases.

First Name	Initial	Last Name		Initials	Subject Number	Center Number	Random Number

City	State	Country		Pincode

Address		Phone	Email

	Private

Additionally you need to input ---

Subject Number

Each participant in the study will have a unique subject number.

Center Number (Site number)

A multi center study will have many site numbers.

Randomization Number

The subject after entry into the study will be randomized to the study drug. He will be assigned a random number that will allot him either the sponsor drug or the active comparator or a placebo.

These above numbers will be reported in the source document.

PATIENT DEMOGRAPHICS

Date of Birth

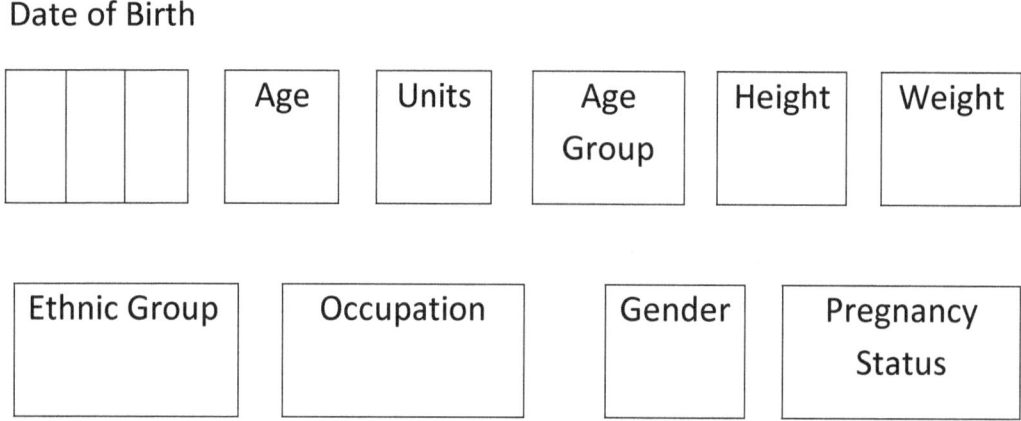

DOB

Input the date of birth in the required format.

Age

This tab is an auto calculated tab. The patient's age is calculated from the date of birth and earliest event onset date if both complete dates are available. In case the complete dates are not available you can calculate from the partial dates and enter the same manually.

Units

The age can be in days, weeks, months and years. This ranges from neonate (days) to elderly (years).

Height

Input the height as reported in the source.

Weight

Input the weight as reported in the source.

Age Groups

The below is an illustration of the age groups

Neonate: 0 – 27 days

Infant: 28 days - 24 months

Child: 2 years - 11 years

Adolescent: 12 - 17 years

Adult: 18 - 64

Elderly: Above 64 years

Ethnic Groups

Caucasian, Afro, Negroid, Asian, Afroasian are examples of some ethnic groups.

Occupation

Select the occupation from the drop down options.

Gender

Male or female. If you enter male the pregnancy tab will be grayed out.

Pregnancy Status

If the gender is female the pregnancy tab remains open.

Choose the appropriate option

Yes: if the patient is pregnant

No: if the patient is female and not pregnant

Unknown: If the patient is female and her pregnancy status is unknown.

PREGNANCY MODULE

Last Menstrual Period	Due Date	Pregnancy Report Type	Weeks at Exposure	Trimester at Exposure

Weeks at Onset	Delivery Date	Type of Delivery	Fetal Outcome	APGAR	BREASTFEED

LMP

Input the date of the last menstrual period if given in the source document.

Due Date

Input the due date (EDD - expected date of delivery) as given in the source document. If not calculate the EDD from the LMP.

Pregnancy report type

This will be either prospective or retrospective.

Weeks At Exposure

The number of gestation weeks at the time of exposure to the suspect drug

Trimester At Exposure

The number of trimester (1, 2 or 3) at the time of exposure to the suspect drug

Weeks At Onset

The number of weeks of pregnancy at the time of onset of the event.

Delivery Date

In the required format

Type Of Delivery

Normal

Cesarean Section

Fetal Outcome

Normal

Abnormal

APGAR Score

The APGAR score ranges from 0 – 10 and is input. It is input in the format 0-10/10 .

The score is input based on the information provided in the source document.

Breastfeed

Breastfeeding or breastfed the baby after birth. Input as

Yes

No

Unknown.

As per the information provided in the source document.

MEDICAL HISTORY

The medical history is a significant input in deciding the causality.

A patient with a medical history of obesity, work stress and diabetes on the suspect drug has an event of myocardial infarction. The medical history of obesity, work stress and diabetes are high risk factors for a heart attack making the suspect drug unlikely related or not related.

A patient with history of drug allergy on a biologic suspect drug develops oral cancer. Taking into consideration the latency and absence of predisposing medical history such as tobacco chewing there could be a possible relationship between the suspect drug and the event.

Presence or absence of medical history is critical in arriving at the causality.

Medical History	Code	Start Date	End Date	Current

Free Text / Notes

Medical History

Input the medical history and code it appropriately. MedDRA is used to code the medical history.

Start Date

Input the start date of the medical history if reported in the source document

End Date: Input the end date of the medical history if reported in the source document

Current Status: Is it ongoing, stopped or unknown as per the source document

Free Text/Notes

In this space write down associated events with the medical history such as hospitalization, complications, surgery.

DEATH MODULE

Date of Death		Autopsy	Results		Death Cause	Code Cause

ADD

Date of Death

Input the date of death

Autopsy

Is the autopsy done? Choose from the below options

Yes

No

Unknown

Results

If autopsy is done what is the status of the autopsy results. Choose

Pending

Available

Death Cause

Input the cause of death as per the source document.

LAB DATA MODULE

Date	Lab Test	Code	Result	Units	Low	High

ADD

You can add more rows to the lab test as required by clicking the ADD button.

Date

Enter the date when the test or lab procedure was done the test was carried out. If complete date is not available enter month or year.

Lab Test

Input the name of the lab test or procedure.

Code

Code the lab test or procedure. MedDRA is used to code the lab test or procedure.

Result

Input the result mentioned in the source document.

Units

Input the units of the result.

Low – High

Input the reference range (normal low - normal high).

RELEVANT TEST

Relevant Test

The relevant test is a free text space which is used to record the results of tests such as MRI (magnetic resonance imaging) CT (computerized tomography) scans and biopsy results. However any test or tests which require more space can be recorded here.

DRUG MODULE

Drug Brand Name
Code To Generic

S	C	T

First Dose	Last Dose	Duration

Form

Taken Previous	Tolerated

Start	End

Dose	Unit

Frequency

TDD

Route of administration

ADD

Indication	Code Indication

ADD

Action Taken	Dechallenge	Rechallenge

Drug Brand Name

Input the brand name of the drug

Generic name

Code to the generic name using the WHO DD (Drug dictionary)

S – Click this tab if the drug is a suspect drug. There can be more than 1 suspect drug. A suspect drug can be a non-company drug.

C - Click this tab if the drug is a concomitant drug. A concomitant drug is one that starts prior to the onset of the adverse events.

T- Click this drug if the drug is a treatment drug. A treatment drug is one whose start date is after the onset of the events and is the drug is given for the treatment of the event.

(For categorization of past, concomitant and treatment drugs follow the guidelines of the sponsor)

First Dose

Start date of the drug

Last Dose

Last dose of the drug

Duration

Difference between the first and last dose

Form

Choose from the drop down options

Tablet, oral solution , capsule, minipill, pill, injection

Taken previous

Has the drug been taken previously by the patient.

Tolerated

When taken previously was it well tolerated or did it have side effects.

Date

Start date and end date of the dosage.

Dose

Dose with unit (Ex: 1 mg, 50mg, 500mg).

Frequency

Frequency of drug administration (OD- once a day, qd: once a day, bid: twice a day, tid: thrice a day. Qid : four times a day, HS: At night).

TDD

Total Daily Dose. If dose and frequency is input the TDD is auto calculated.

Route of administration

Oral, inhalation, transdermal, subcutaneous, intramuscular.

By clicking ADD you get additional dosage regimen tab.

Indication

The disease for which the suspect drug has been started to treat.

Code the indication using MedDRA.

By clicking ADD you get additional indication tab.

Action Taken

- Dose continued (If the drug is ongoing)
- Dose reduced (If the dose is decreased after the start of the event)
- Dose increased (If the dose is increased after the start of the event)
- Drug withdrawn (If the drug is discontinued)
- Temporarily discontinued (If the drug is stopped with a plan to restart)

Dechallenge

If an event or events resolve, resolve with sequelae or are resolving after Dose reduction, Drug withdrawal (temporary or permanent)

Rechallenge

If the event or events reappear on restart of the drug. A rechallenge is only possible if a dechallenge is positive.

EVENT MODULE.

Reported Verbatim	Modify	Code The Event

D	LT	H/POH	DIS	CA	IME	OTHER

Start Date	End Date	Duration	Outcome

AESI

Reported Verbatim

The term reported in the source document for the event should be input here. This may not be exactly the codable term. It can be a diagnosis, symptom or sign or an abnormal lab test. It may also be a short description of the event rather than the medical term or diagnosis.

Modify

This is a free text space where the reported verbatim term or phrase can be modified into a codable medical term.

Code The Event

The event term can be auto – coded. If it does not get auto-coded then do a manual coding. Use MEdDRA for coding the event.

The second row represents the seriousness criteria. If the event is serious then at least one of the below seriousness criteria has to be ticked.

D - Death

LT – Life - threatening

H – Hospitalisation

POH – Prolongation of hospitalization

Dis – Disability (temporary or permanent)

CA – Congenital anomaly

IME – Important medical event (The event may be in the IME list)

Other – If the event is not any of these seriousness criteria then this tab can be ticked if the event is medically significant) serous as per medical judgment).

Start Date

Input the start date

End Date

Input the end date

Duration

Duration of the event is auto calculated if both start and stop dates are full dates.

Outcome: Outcome can be

Resolved

Resolved with sequelae

Resolving

Not resolved

Unknown

Not applicable : Sometimes the outcome of non – clinical events such as drug exposure during pregnancy, drug exposure in utero, medication error are marked as not applicable.

AESI – Adverse events of special interest. These are specific to the drug and specific to the sponsor. So you need to know the AESI for your company drugs to mark this tab.

CAUSALITY AND EXPECTEDNESS

Event	Reporter	Company	CCDS	SPC	IB

Causality

Binary causality

This type of causality has only 2 options

a. Related – The event is related to the drug

b. Not related – The event is not related to the drug

Reporter's causality

The reporter assesses various parameters including whether the medical history , concomitant drugs or drug – drug interaction might be a cause of the event. The reporter may use terms such as definitely related, highly probably related, probably related, possibly related all of which translate to Related in the binary system. After evaluation of the causative factors the reporter may assess the causality as not related. The reporter's causality should be input as reported in the source document.

Company causality

At medical review the reviewer assesses the company causality and inputs in the database for each event.

Expectedness

At medical review the reviewer checks for the event in CCDS, SmPC and the IB.

If the event term or the synonym is present in the RSI (CCDS, SmPC or IB) the event is listed. If it is not present in the RSI the event is unexpected.

The IB is the only document for drugs which are still in the clinical trial phase.

DECHALLENGE AND RECHALLENGE

Event

DC	RC

Dechallenge

When a suspect drug is discontinued either temporarily or permanently and the event resolves, resolves with sequelae or is resolving then dechallenge is positive for the event. If the event is not resolved then the dechallenge is negative.

Rechallenge

Rechallenge is only possible if dechallenge is positive. If the suspect drug is reintroduced and the event reappears then dechallenge is positive. If the event does not reappear then the dechallenge is negative.

DC and RC

Dechallenge and rechallenge should be assessed for each event and input.

NARRATIVE

Sender's Comment

Case Analysis Section

The Case Analysis section of the Case Analysis tab enables you to enter narrative information about the adverse event. The following is an illustration of the Case Analysis section.

After the narrative is written the sender's comment (PSUR comment) has to be written. This comment appears in the line listing. It contains vital information in a snapshot and allows the physician to assess the causality quickly. Hence it should be written by an expert. Generally **the sender's comment** starts with relevant medical history and then goes on to list the adverse events that have occurred after initiating the suspect and co-suspect drugs. The latency is an important input in deciding the causality. It then mentions whether the patient was hospitalized and received medical or surgical treatment. The action taken with the suspect and co-suspect drugs and the outcomes of the events. Finally the reporter's causality if available is input.

ORACLE ARGUS OVERVIEW

GENERAL INFORMATION

PATIENT MODULE

PRODUCT MODULE

EVENT MODULE

ANALYSIS TAB

ARGUS OVERVIEW

Below are additional fields which you may come across when you work on Oracle ARGUS. These have to be read in context with the generic database already described.

<u>The Work Flow</u>

Book In

Case Process

Medical Review

Distribution

Moving the case to the next level is called Route.

After Book In the case is Routed to Case Process.

After Case processing the case is routed to Medical Review.

After Medical Review the case is Routed to Distribution.

From distribution the case is submitted to different regulatory authorities. The case is submitted to those countries where it is marketed.

Book In: In this step the case is created. The case is created only if it qualifies as a valid case.

Case Process: In this step the details of the reporter, drug, and events are input.

Medical Review: In this step causality, listedness and analaysis modules are completed. Event coding is checked for accuracy.

GENERAL INFORMATION

You need to select the reporter's occupation from a drop down.

You can identify a primary reporter. Only one primary reporter is allowed.

If the reporter is a healthcare professional select Yes, No, or unknown from a drop down lost as appropriate.

Auto-population of literature information is possible. Open the literature reference dialog and select the specified reference. The details of the of the selected literature information are auto populated to corresponding fields in the literature information.

PATIENT MODULE

In addition to patient information and details patient tab includes medical history and death modules.

Medical History.

After encoding the medical history you can do the following actions.

Copy: Copy a row.

Add: Add a row (to add another history).

Delete: Delete a row (if you have added a wrong history).

Up and Down: Move a row up or down (if you want to arrange it in any particular order).

Death Module

Date of Death

Autopsy Done

Report Available

Cause of Death

Description as reported	Encode

If Autopsy Done is entered as No or Unknown the Autopsy Results Available is auto populated to No.

The following actions are available in the Death Module

Encode: Encodes the description as reported

Add: You can add the row of Cause of Death and Description as reported

Delete: You can delete the row

Up and Down: You can move the row up and down.

PRODUCT MODULE

In the product module you can input the name of the drug and information about the dosage regimen and indication. You can choose to list the drug as a suspect, concomitant or treatment drug.

In the case of a clinical trial blinded study, the blinded name is coded (Ex: sponsor drug name vs placebo; suspect drug name vs comparator drug name).

In addition to the drug view, vaccine or device views are available in the product module. However the default view is the drug view.

How to input the drug name

First Line   - Drug Name

Second Line - Generic Name

In the first line input the brand (trade name). In the second line input the generic name (active ingredient).

Drug Code / Medicinal Product ID

You can search using either the drug code or the medicinal product identification number. The default option is the Drug Code.

Trade Name / Active Ingredient Name

You can search using either the brand (trade) name or the active ingredient name. The default option is set to the Brand Name.

Formulation

You can search the drug based on the drug formulation.

Formulation The form in which the drug was administered (liquid, tablet, capsule, etc.)

Country

You can search the drug based on the country where the drug was marketed.

Adding Additional Rows

Click the Add button to add more rows.

Deleting Entries

Click the button, to highlight the row for removal.

Sorting the Entries

The Lab data can be sorted in chronological order by Date of the Test and alphabetically by the Test Name

The Lab Data section provides data about lab test and test results. The maximum number of lab test data on the Case Form is 2000.

Drug Search

You can search for the drug in two ways

- WHO Drug Search

- Product Search

> How to conduct a WHO Drug Browser Search

1. Select the Encode button to open the WHO Drug Coding.

2. You need to enter the following features of the drug and click Search.

   o Brand name
   o Formulation
   o Strength
   o Sales Country Code of the drug

> How to conduct a search using Product Search

Enter the name of the product using the Select button. You can enter a product name partially also. Then press TAB. This displays the Product Selection dialog.

If the study is blinded, the blinded name of the study is displayed.

You can click the below click boxes in the ARGUS product module

Outside Therapeutic Range: Tick this click box if the drug dose is outside the therapeutic range.

Abuse: Tick this click box if the patient has abused the drug. Opiates are commonly abused drugs. If drugs are taken as a result of psychological dependence rather than for the treatment of a medical condition this results in drug abuse.

Overdose: Tick this click box if the patient has taken an overdose of the product.

Interaction: Tick this click box If the drug is part of drug-drug interaction.

Tampering: Tick this click box if the drug has been tampered with before it was used.

In the following sections you need to select or input appropriately

Parent Route of Administration: You need to select the route of administration for the parent in case of a baby report.

Accidental Exposure. You can select the type of accidental exposure from a list.

Taken previously / Tolerated: This refers to whether the drug has been used by the patient previously and if Yes whether it had been well tolerated. Input the appropriate response.

Action Taken: Select the appropriate action taken from the list. The action taken ranges from Dose not changed to Drug withdrawn. If you select Dose Increased or No Change, the dechallenge and rechallenge fields will be greyed out.

Drug Batch Details

Package ID: You need to enter the package identification number.

Batch/Lot Number: You need to enter the batch and/or lot number(s).

Expiry Date: You need to enter the date of expiry of the drug. You can enter a partial date.

In the ARGUS product module you can switch views by clicking the additional product tab.

The following are the icons that represent the different views.

VC- Vaccine view selected

DR- Drug view selected

DV- Device view selected

Study Drug

For a non-configured study a study drug can be entered in a case. You can mark a current product as a study drug.

To make a suspect product as a study drug

1. Right click on any suspect product in the case.
2. Select Make Study Drug. Select the study therapy from a drop down list.

   This field – Make Study Drug – is only for non-configured study. If the study is blinded, this field is disabled. The drugs listed in the drop down list are based on the Study ID selected in the General Module.

Study Drug is a read-only field that contains the product name selected by the user from a drop down list which contains drugs based on the study ID. This field is only for unblinded (previously blinded but currently blind broken by the sponsor or the investigator) or not blinded clinical trial cases only.

Quality Control

Argus has specific module for product quality complaint. You can enter quality control information by clicking the QC Info button and entering the appropriate information in the Quality Control dialog.

- QC department reference number for the analysis.
- QC Sent Date
- Date Returned
- CID Number: Control Identification Number.
- PCID Number: Enter the Product Control Identification Number.
- QC Result Date Enter the date the result of the analysis was received by the QC department.
- QC Result Enter a text explanation as necessary. Use the zoom icon to open the zoom notes and view or edit the text.
- QC comment: Enter any comment relating to the analysis.

EVENT MODULE

In the event module you can

- ➤ Code adverse events
- ➤ Input the criteria for the seriousness
- ➤ Review the auto input of event listedness

Code Events (Event coding section)

Description as Reported: Enter the verbatim from the source document as reported by the reporter.

Description to be coded: The verbatim term is auto copied under Description to be Coded.

If necessary, the verbatim term can be modified in this field. For example,

The reported verbatim is – Red itchy rash

The options available for coding are – Erythematous rash and Pruritic rash.

So the reported verbatim can possibly split to –

Red rash

Itchy rash

The reported verbatim may be modified appropriately to reflect the medical term.

The reported verbatim is – Pus collection

The option for coding is – Abscess

So the reported verbatim may be modified to Abscess

The reported verbatim is - Problem with swallowing

The option for coding is – Dysphagia

The reported verbatim may be modified to Difficulty in swallowing

Using the MedDRA Browser

The MedDRA application searches the term dictionary for a match at the Lower level term or at the Synonym level. If a match is found, the following fields are automatically populated: Term code, Preferred Term, Included Term, High Level Term, Group Term and Body System/SOC.

With MedDRA (Medical Dictionary of regulatory authority) hierarchy of coding is seen as below:

SOC – System Organ Class

HLGT – High Level Group Term

HLT – High Level Term

PT – Preferred term

LLT – Lower Level Term

Once the LLT is matched with the reported verbatim and the appropriate code is selected the hierarchy is uneditable.

More often than not you will get the exact match as there are more than 70,000 lower level terms in MedDRA. In some cases when you cannot get the exact match to the reported verbatim or the modified term you need to exercise medical judgment to select the appropriate code.

You get the option of choosing from a list of synonyms generated by the system.

All these make sure that the event coding is just perfect!

Some databases also have option of coding with ART. The administrator can set the dictionary you prefer to code with.

Seriousness Criteria: Tick the click boxes to indicate the seriousness criteria.

Diagnosis - Relationship: Click the Relationships tab to see the Diagnosis-Event Relationships. Here you can club symptoms to the diagnoses.

Encode : Click this button to search for the term entered under Event Description. The entered term is checked in the MedDRA dictionary.

Dropped from Study due to Event: For clinical trial cases only. Select this check box if the subject was dropped from the study due to this adverse event.

Term Highlighted by Reporter: Make the appropriate selection to indicate whether the person reporting the event considered it to be serious. Selecting Yes does not mark this case as Serious automatically.

Associated with Rechallenge : Only opens if a suspect drug has be restarted for rechallenge.

Enter Hospitalization Details

1. Select the Hospitalized check box under Seriousness Criteria.
2. The form for Hospitalization Details appears. Enter the first and last date of the hospitalization. Partial dates are allowed. The duration is auto calculated.

Change Event Outcome

When the Event outcome on the Events Tab is changed and the event outcome and case outcome don't match the following message pops up in ARGUS.

Case outcome may no longer match events.

Diagnosis-Event

You can club different events and link them to a single diagnosis. The case must contain at minimum of two events and one diagnosis. The symptoms are indented and associated to the diagnosis.

This makes the medical review more meaningful. For instance you can club the events rigidity and tremors and difficulty in walking under the diagnosis of Parkinson's disease.

This also helps in the line listing as it reports only the diagnosis.

 This feature aids significantly in the interpretation and review of individual case reports. It is also useful in summary reports as it enables the reporting of diagnoses only, while retaining database records of individual event terms.

Click the Relationships button in the Event Information section of the Event tab to open the Diagnosis-Event relationship

.

Event Assessment Tab

In the event Assessment section the following are displayed

Causality of each event

- Reported Causaity: As reported by the reporter in the source document.
- As determined causality (company causality): Causality assessed by the medical reviewer considering the medical history, latency, drug - drug interaction, drug disease interaction and other possible contributing factors.

Listedness (expectedness) of each event

Oracle ARGUS auto checks the listedness of every event. All events are compared with the listed terms in sponsor drug RSI – CCDS, SmPC and IB.

Recalculate: If new events are entered or click the Recalculate button. In case the listedness has been you need to recheck the auto- populated listedness.

In the event assessment tab you can input the causality and enter the listedness.

Event	Reporter Causality	As Determined Causality	CCDS

			SPC

			IB

On clicking the Recalculate button the listedness is auto calculated by the system.

If the auto listedness is changed a case justification box pops up. You need to enter the rationale for changing the listedness.

On clicking the Recalculate button the system does not recalculate listedness when the event assessment listedness already has a case justification either manually written or generated by the system.

ANALYSIS TAB

In addition to the narrative and sender's comment (PSUR comment), the analysis tab also has information required for generating the MedWatch 3500A, BfArM, and AFSSaPS reports.

Using Auto Narrative Templates

You can select an Auto Narrative template for the Narrative, Case Comment and evaluation. It is possible to edit the auto narrative.

Viewing Differences in Case Narratives

The system enables you to view the differences in case comments from previously locked versions of the case. To view these differences, you need to click the Show Difference button in the Case Comments section.

- Displays the differences in red with a strike out and a yellow highlight.
- Displays additions to the narrative in black with green highlights.

- The Narrative is read-only.

Case Analysis Fields

Narrative - Can be auto generated. It is editable. The narrative is printed on expedited reports.

Case Comment - You can enter comments in this area. Comments appear on certain expedited reports

Evaluation Comment - Enter an evaluation comment that takes into consideration similar events that have occurred in the past

Company Comment - Enter comments in this area. This information does not appear on expedited reports.

Abbreviated Narrative - Enter brief comments in this field. This item maps only to the PSUR report.

For more details of The Advanced Pharmacovigilance Database

Visit www.gipv.net

Online Pharmacovigilance.

- ➢ How to do a DUPLICATE Search
- ➢ How to set up a PQC
- ➢ What is a biologic, latency, causality, adverse event as per GVP
- ➢ E2B Fields & Conventions
- ➢ Chronic alcoholic on suspect drug develops pain. He consults a medic and is diagnosed with pancreatitis. If you miss to input the medical history in the database will this be a critical error?
- ➢ All about PV Online—One stop resource for PV.

www.gipv.net

PROFESSIONAL PHARMACOVIGILANCE CERTIFICATION

Titles By Dr. Ravi N Humbarwadi

Pharmacovigilance : Principles and Practice.

Concepts of champions (Kindle and Amazon) – Deals with Long Term
Management Success.

Pharmacoepidemiology

Pharmacovigilance and Pharmacoepidemiology

This Book Is Sponsored by

www.gipv.net

Pharmacovigilance Online

INITIAL CASE ENTRY - CASE PROCESSING - ACTION TAKEN -
EXPECTEDNESS/LISTEDNESS

NARRATIVE WRITING - COMPANY COMMENT - CASE STUDIES -
PREGNANCY CASES

www.gipv.net

Oracle Argus Simplified – Advance PV Database – E2B – ICH GCP

E- learning. Skill Testing. Certification.